Eye Ex

Seniors

A Proven Way to Improve
Vision, Reduce Eye Strain and
your Overall Eye Health Safely
and Effectively

Max J. Hudson

Contents

CHAPTER ONE

Introduction to Eye Exercises

Eye exercises are a set of techniques and activities designed to improve and maintain the health and functionality of the eyes. These exercises are designed to improve visual acuity, strengthen eye muscles, and decrease eye strain. They are especially important for seniors because age-related changes might damage eyesight, making preventive eye care vital.

Why are Eye Exercises Important for Seniors?

Age-Related Vision Changes: As people age, their eyes undergo a variety of changes, including decreasing pupil size, decreased tear production, and a gradual loss of the capacity to focus on close objects. Eye workouts can help offset these changes and keep your vision in good shape.

Preventing Eye Conditions: Seniors are more likely than younger people to acquire eye conditions such as cataracts, glaucoma, and macular degeneration. Regular eye workouts can help to reduce the risk of certain disorders or decrease their growth.

Reducing Digital Eye Strain: In today's digital world, seniors may spend more time looking at displays, which might result in digital eye strain or computer vision syndrome. Eye exercises can help reduce the pain caused by prolonged screen use.

Improving Quality of Life: Seniors need good vision to preserve their independence, enjoy hobbies, and participate in daily activities. By sustaining visual function, eye exercises can contribute to an improved quality of life

Benefits of Eye Exercises for seniors

Eye workouts can improve your capacity to see minute details, making it simpler to read, recognize faces, and accomplish other daily duties.

Eye Muscle Control: These exercises improve the muscles involved for focusing, tracking objects, and maintaining eye alignment, lowering the likelihood of strabismus (crossed eyes) and amblyopia (lazy eye).

Reduced Eye weariness: Exercises that relax the eye muscles and reduce weariness can help seniors who suffer from eye strain from reading, using digital gadgets, or doing close-up work.

Improved Peripheral Vision: Certain eye exercises can assist to extend the field of vision, which is extremely important for seniors when driving or navigating their surroundings.

How to Do Eye Exercises Safely and Effectively:

Consult an Eye Care Professional: Before beginning any eye exercise plan, speak with an eye care professional, such as an optometrist or ophthalmologist. They can evaluate your vision and provide advice geared to your individual needs.

Maintain a Routine: Establish a regular routine for completing eye workouts. Consistency is essential for reaching and maintaining achievements.

Warm-up: Begin by gently pressing your palms together to generate heat. For a few seconds, cup your warm palms over your closed eyes to calm them.

Practice Eye Yoga: To enhance focus and flexibility, use activities such as palming (covering your closed eyes with your palms), blinking quickly, and focusing on distant and near things.

Massage the area around your eyes with your fingertips in moderate circular strokes. This can assist to reduce stress and promote blood circulation.

Use Visual Aids: To strengthen your long-distance vision, use tools such as eye charts or focus on distant objects. To improve your near eyesight, practice reading fine text.

Be patient: It may take some time for you to improve. Consistent practice over several weeks or months is often required to see major gains in vision.

Avoid Strain: If a workout causes discomfort or strain, stop immediately and visit your eye doctor.

Finally, eye exercises can help seniors maintain and improve their vision as they get older. Seniors can benefit from greater visual acuity, reduced eye strain, and a higher overall quality of life by performing these exercises safely and on a regular basis. Before beginning any new fitness program, especially one for your eyes, always consult with a healthcare practitioner.

Types of Eye Exercises

Here are some eye exercises that seniors can implement into their daily routine to improve and maintain their vision:

Focusing (near and far):

Focus on a small object (such as a pen) at arm's length for a few seconds.

Then, for a few seconds, move your gaze to an object in the distance (across the room or outside).

To strengthen your eye's capacity to shift focus, alternate between near and far things.

The Eighth Figure:

Consider an eight turned on its side (the infinity sign).

Trace the shape with your eyes, beginning at the center and progressing along the lines.

This workout improves eye coordination and flexibility.

Palming:

To generate heat, vigorously rub your palms together.

Cup your warm palms over your closed eyes without applying any pressure.

Take a few deep breaths and relax. Visualize darkness as you do this.

Palming can help with eye strain and relaxation.

Blinking:

Blinking is a natural exercise, but it must be done deliberately.

Blink several times quickly, then close your eyes for a few seconds.

This moisturizes the eyes and relieves dryness and inflammation.

20-20-20 Rule:

When working on a computer or reading for an extended period of time, take a 20-second break and look at anything at least 20 feet away every 20 minutes.

This guideline helps to relieve digital eye strain and relax the eye muscles.

Zooming:

Place your thumb about 10 inches in front of your face and sit comfortably.

For a few seconds, concentrate on your thumb.

Bring your thumb closer to your nose while maintaining your focus.

Then, gradually return it to its original place.

Repeat this practice several times to enhance your capacity to focus.

Refocusing:

Choose two objects at varying distances, such as a book and a faraway tree.

Alternate your sight between the two objects, focusing for a few seconds on each.

This practice trains your eyes to quickly alter their focus.

Yoga for the Eyes:

Eye yoga movements include rotating your eyes in a circular manner, moving them up and down, and side to side.

These movements aid in the improvement of eye mobility and the reduction of strain.

Exercises with an Eye Chart:

Using an eye chart, practice reading small print or letters from various distances.

Regularly exercising your eyes with different font sizes might help improve visual acuity.

Exercises in Convergence:

Place your finger about an inch in front of your nose.

Focus on your finger, then move it slowly towards your nose while maintaining focus.

This exercise can aid in the improvement of convergence, which is necessary for near vision.

Keep in mind to do these exercises lightly and without tension. Consult an eye care specialist if you are experiencing discomfort or worsening of any eye issue. Incorporating these activities into a daily routine will help seniors maintain good eye health and visual function.

CHAPTER TWO

How to Do Eye Exercises

Here are specific instructions for some common types of eye exercises:

Palming:

- Locate a quiet, comfortable spot to sit.
- To generate heat, vigorously rub your hands together.
- Gently cup your warm palms over your closed eyes without placing any pressure on them.
- Make sure no light penetrates your eyes; your palms should provide a dark, relaxing environment.

- Take several deep, steady breaths and close your eyes for 1-2 minutes.
- While palming, imagine a relaxing environment or a blank, dark space.
- Remove your palms from your eyes slowly, blinking several times to acclimatize to the light.
- Palming helps to relax eye muscles and reduces eye strain.

Exercise in Blinking:

- Sit or stand up straight and keep your eyes open.
- Blink your eyes 10 to 15 times quickly.

- Close your eyes and rest them for roughly 20 seconds after fast blinking.
- Rep this cycle 3–4 times.

Benefits: Rapid blinking followed by brief resting periods helps moisturize and reduce dryness in the eyes, which is especially beneficial for those who spend a lot of time looking at digital devices.

Changing the focus:

- Find a seated position that is comfortable for you.
- Extend your arm and lift your thumb, concentrating your sight on it.

- Bring your thumb closer to your nose while maintaining attention.
- When maintaining attention gets difficult, carefully slide your thumb away from your nose.
- Repeat this exercise 10-15 times while keeping your thumb clear and focused.

Benefits: Focus shifting exercises enhance your capacity to switch between near and far things, increasing your general eye flexibility.

Close-up Focus:

- Sit or stand comfortably, with a clear view of a distant

object and a close-up book or text.

- For a few seconds, fix your eyes on the faraway object.
- Then, for a few seconds, turn your attention to the close-up text.
- For 1-2 minutes, alternate your focus between the distant object and the close-up text.

Benefits: This exercise improves accommodation (the capacity of the eye to focus on different distances), which reduces eye strain while switching between near and far work.

Rolling the eyes:

- Sit with your back straight and comfortable.
- Take a step forward.
- Roll your eyes slowly in a clockwise manner for 10-15 seconds.
- Then, for 10-15 seconds, roll them counterclockwise.
- This exercise should be repeated 2-3 times in each direction.
- Eye rolling improves eye movement and can reduce sensations of eye tiredness.

Figure 8: Eye Movement

- Consider a massive figure eight (infinity symbol) in front of you.

- Follow the imaginary figure eight pattern with your eyes without moving your head.
- Trace the figure eight in one direction for 30 seconds, then switch directions for another 30 seconds.

This practice improves eye coordination and flexibility.

Remember to practice these exercises lightly, without straining your eyes. Stop immediately and consult an eye care specialist if you develop discomfort or pain while exercising. Furthermore, consistency is essential. Over time, regular practice of these exercises might lead to improved results in terms of preserving and improving your eye health.

How Often to Do Eye Exercises

The frequency of eye workouts for seniors can vary depending on their demands and level of comfort. However, incorporating eye exercises into their daily routine is a basic guideline for how often seniors should do them to reap the maximum benefits. Here's a more in-depth breakdown:

Daily Practice: To get the most out of eye exercises, seniors should do them every day. Maintaining healthy vision and strengthening eye muscles require consistency.

Short Sessions: You don't have to devote long periods of time to eye workouts. Short sessions of 5 to 10 minutes in length, repeated throughout the day, can be beneficial. This can aid in the prevention of eye strain and weariness.

Variety is Important: Instead than doing the same exercise over and again, switch it up. This helps to use different eye muscles and keeps you from becoming bored.

Pay Attention to Your Eyes: Take note of how your eyes feel throughout and after the workouts. Take a pause if you start to experience any discomfort, strain, or exhaustion. Exercising your eyes too much can be harmful.

Consult an Eye Care Professional:

Working with an optometrist or ophthalmologist to develop a personalized eye exercise plan tailored to your unique needs is critical. Based on your eye health and any underlying issues, they can advise you on the best exercises and frequency.

Remember that the purpose of eye exercises is to progressively maintain and enhance eye health.

It could take some time before you notice major changes in your eyesight or less eye strain. Be patient and consistent, and always seek the advice of a healthcare practitioner on the best workouts and program for your specific circumstances.

Tips for Getting the Most Out of Eye Exercises

In order to include eye exercises into your daily routine and maximize their effectiveness, you must be committed and consistent. Here are some pointers to make the most of your eye exercises:

Make a Schedule: Schedule your eye exercises for a certain time each day. Consistency is essential for seeing results.

Make a calm Space: Locate a calm, well-lit space free of distractions where you may conduct your eye exercises comfortably.

Warm-up: To relax your eye muscles, begin your eye training regimen with a short warm-up. This can be accomplished by gently rubbing your palms together to create warmth, then cupping your heated palms over your closed eyes for a few seconds.

Maintain a Relaxed Posture: Maintain a relaxed posture throughout the workouts. Tension in your body can reduce the efficiency of your workouts.

Deep, controlled breathing can help you relax and lower overall stress, both of which can benefit your eye health.

Follow Professional Guidance: If an eye care doctor has given you a specific set of exercises, carefully follow their directions. They can design workouts to meet your specific requirements.

Be patient: Vision improvement may not occur immediately. Allow your eyes to adjust and strengthen. Significant outcomes may take several weeks or months to appear.

Gradually increase the difficulty of an exercise if it becomes too easy. Increase the difficulty gradually to keep your eyes engaged.

Use Visual Aids: To make your practice more exciting and effective, incorporate resources such as eye charts, near and far objects, or specialist apps created for vision workouts.

Maintain a notebook to document your daily exercises and any changes in your vision. This can help you stay motivated while also providing useful insights into your progress.

Hydration and nutrition: Keep hydrated because dehydration can cause dry eyes and discomfort. A healthy diet high in antioxidants and nutrients such as vitamins A, C, and E can help with overall eye health.

Stop immediately and consult with your eye care provider if any workout produces pain, discomfort, or increasing vision difficulties. Safety should always come first.

Regular Eye checks: Continue to see your eye care specialist for regular checks to monitor your eye health and make necessary adjustments to your workouts.

Maintain a cheerful Attitude: Maintain a cheerful attitude. Believing in the benefits of your exercises can have a psychological impact on the improvement of your vision.

Along with your activities, consider additional lifestyle adjustments such as decreasing screen time, adopting suitable lighting, and taking regular breaks whether working on a computer or reading.

Remember that the effectiveness of eye exercises varies from person to person, and they should not be used in place of medical therapy for certain eye disorders. For the best results, always consult with an eye care specialist before beginning any new eye exercise plan, and always follow their advice.

CHAPTER THREE

Common Eye Problems in seniors

Certainly, the following are some of the most prevalent eye disorders that seniors face:

Presbyopia is a natural age-related disorder in which the lens of the eye loses flexibility, making it harder to concentrate on close objects. This illness often manifests itself around the age of 40 and worsens with age. Presbyopia is frequently treated with reading glasses or bifocals.

Cataracts are a clouding of the natural lens of the eye that causes blurred vision and reduced visual clarity. Because of the aging process, seniors are more prone to cataracts, and surgery to remove the hazy lens and replace it with an artificial lens is a popular treatment.

Glaucoma is a category of eye illnesses that damage the optic nerve, often as a result of increasing eye pressure. It is the major cause of blindness in the elderly. Regular eye examinations are essential for early detection and treatment, which may include eye drops, surgery, or laser treatments.

AMD (Age-Related Macular Degeneration): AMD is a progressive disorder that affects the macula, the center region of the retina that is important for sharp, central vision. It is a leading cause of severe vision loss in elderly persons and can cause blurred or distorted vision.

Diabetic Retinopathy: Diabetes-affected seniors are at risk of developing diabetic retinopathy, a disorder in which high blood sugar levels damage the blood vessels in the retina. If not treated adequately with medicine or laser treatments, it might result in visual loss.

Dry Eye Syndrome: As people age, their tear production decreases, resulting in dry eyes. This can result in pain, a burning sensation, and vision issues. Dry eye is frequently treated with artificial tears and lifestyle changes.

Floaters and flashes of light: Seniors may notice floaters (small, black spots or cobweb-like shapes) and flashes of light in their vision. These are normally harmless, but an eye doctor should be consulted to rule out any serious underlying disorders.

Retinal Detachment: Seniors have a slightly increased risk of retinal detachment, which occurs when the retina detaches from the back of the eye. This might result in sudden visual loss, necessitating rapid surgical intervention.

Ptosis is a disorder in which the top eyelid droops and partially covers the eye. It can arise as a result of aging or other underlying medical issues and, if severe, can impair vision.

Refractive Errors: Seniors' vision may shift due to nearsightedness (myopia), farsightedness (hyperopia), or astigmatism. These problems are treatable with glasses, contact lenses, or refractive surgery.

Regular eye exams are necessary for seniors in order to detect and treat common eye issues as early as possible. Early intervention and therapy can aid in the management of various disorders, as well as the preservation or improvement of seniors' vision and general quality of life.

How Eye Exercises Can Help with Common Eye Problems

Eye exercises can help improve eyesight and alleviate the symptoms of common eye disorders that seniors may encounter. While they may not heal certain disorders completely, they can assist improve visual function and decrease discomfort. Here are some ways that eye workouts might help with common eye disorders in seniors:

Presbyopia:

Presbyopia is a natural age-related disorder in which the lens of the eye loses flexibility, making it harder to concentrate on close objects.

Changes in focus between near and distant objects can assist strengthen the flexibility of the eye's focusing muscles.

Accommodative exercises, such as focusing on a close item and then a distant one, can assist seniors in more quickly adjusting their concentration.

Digital Vision Strain:

Prolonged screen use can cause digital eye strain, which manifests as symptoms such as dryness, eye tiredness, and blurred vision.

Eye exercises such as the 20-20-20 rule (taking a 20-second break every 20 minutes to look at something 20 feet away) can help relax eye muscles and lessen strain caused by gazing at screens.

Eyes that are dry:

Dry eyes are common in seniors as a result of decreased tear production and environmental variables.

Blinking activities, such as repeatedly blinking in a sequence, can help disseminate tears evenly across the eyes and relieve dryness.

Flashes and floaters:

The gel-like substance in the eye (vitreous) can change as we age, causing the perception of floaters or flashes of light.

Moving your eyes in different directions can assist redistribute the vitreous fluid and reduce the perception of floaters.

Glaucoma:

Glaucoma is a disorder characterized by increasing intraocular pressure, which causes optic nerve damage and vision loss.

According to some research, daily eye exercises that enhance blood circulation and lower intraocular pressure can potentially supplement glaucoma treatment.

AMD (Age-Related Macular Degeneration):

Because of damage to the macula, the core region of the retina, AMD causes central vision loss.

While eye workouts cannot correct AMD, they can increase peripheral vision and the capacity to utilise the retina's remaining healthy components effectively.

Astigmatism:

Astigmatism is a refractive error that results from an unevenly shaped cornea or lens, resulting in blurred or distorted vision.

Specific eye workouts that target the muscles that control the shape of the lens or cornea can help lessen visual disruptions caused by astigmatism.

Strabismus and Lazy Eye (Amblyopia):

Amblyopia (lazy eye) and strabismus (crossed eyes) are both conditions characterized by an imbalance in the use of the eyes.

Eye exercises that encourage the use of both eyes simultaneously and enhance eye coordination might help alleviate these issues, especially if begun early in childhood.

It is crucial to remember that the effectiveness of eye exercises varies depending on the individual and the condition. Seniors should see an eye care specialist before beginning any eye training plan to establish the most effective activities for their unique needs. Regular eye exams are also essential for monitoring eye health and detecting any problems early. While eye exercises can help to keep your eyes healthy, they should be done in conjunction with medical advice and treatments from eye care specialists.

Dear Reader,

Thank you from the depths of our hearts for choosing to explore the pages of "Eye Exercises for Seniors." Your commitment to better vision and well-being inspires us.

In these pages, we've shared the gift of clearer sight and improved eye health. We hope these exercises bring brightness to your world, allowing you to relish every detail life has to offer.

Your dedication to self-care and your eagerness to learn is truly remarkable. We're excited for you to embark on this journey towards stronger, healthier eyes.

As you delve into this book, remember that every exercise is a step toward sharper vision and a more vibrant life. We're grateful to be a part of your quest for improved eyesight, and we can't wait to see the positive changes it brings to your life.

Wishing you clear vision, endless vitality, and countless beautiful moments ahead.

With heartfelt gratitude,

Max J. Hudson

Printed in Great Britain
by Amazon

42864913R00030